"Having watched Alexis interact with clients from a diversity of backgrounds over the three decades we have known each other, I have always been impressed by her gentle confidence and natural inquisitiveness. A true healer who knows and implements both the science and art of medicine, she has always impressed me by her desire to break new boundaries and think beyond ordinary paradigms."

–Deepak Chopra, MD

"For years, Jin Shin self-help has been my saving grace, pulling me and even my bandmates through a range of crises, from food poisoning on a twelve-hour flight to South America to a flu passing through our band bus. Once one becomes empowered by Jin Shin self-help, life starts afresh!"

–Maria Schneider, Grammy Award winner and leader of Maria Schneider Orchestra

"The Art of Jin Shin is an energetic healing modality that is a powerful complementary practice to Western medicine."

–Maurice Preter, MD, integrative neuropsychiatrist

"The Art of Jin Shin is a powerful self-help tool that can be extremely helpful for dancers, as the unblocking and release of energy can aid in injury prevention and more rapid healing of injuries."

—Nikki Feirt Atkins, founder and producing artistic director, American Dance Machine for the Twenty-First Century

"I have been seeing Alexis Brink for over fifteen years, and whenever I'm in New York City I make sure to get a treatment. I always leave a session more energized, yet calmer, and am better able to go about my day in a peaceful, joyful state. Alexis is a first-rate healer/practitioner and I highly recommend her to anyone suffering with a particular health issue or anxiety issue, or those who simply want to be at their optimal level of being!"

—Debbie Gibson, singer, recording artist

"I knew nothing of the Art of Jin Shin before I met Alexis Brink—she has made a believer out of me. My stressed-out body found calm and my exhaustion gave way to energy. This ancient practice should be a prescription for all women who do too much."

—Deborah Roberts, journalist and mother

HEALING

AT YOUR

FINGERTIPS

QUICK FIXES
from *THE ART OF JIN SHIN*

HEALING
······· AT YOUR ·······
FINGERTIPS

ALEXIS BRINK

TILLER PRESS

New York   London   Toronto   Sydney   New Delhi

TILLER PRESS

An Imprint of Simon & Schuster, Inc.
1230 Avenue of the Americas
New York, NY 10020

First Tiller Press trade paperback edition December 2020

TILLER PRESS and colophon are trademarks of Simon & Schuster, Inc.

For information about special discounts for bulk purchases, please contact Simon & Schuster Special Sales at 1-866-506-1949 or business@simonandschuster.com.

The Simon & Schuster Speakers Bureau can bring authors to your live event. For more information or to book an event, contact the Simon & Schuster Speakers Bureau at 1-866-248-3049 or visit our website at www.simonspeakers.com.

Interior design by Jennifer Chung

Manufactured in the United States of America

3 5 7 9 10 8 6 4 2

Library of Congress Cataloging-in-Publication Data

Names: Brink, Alexis, author.
Title: Healing at your fingertips : quick fixes from the art of Jin Shin / by Alexis Brink.
Description: First Tiller Press trade paperback edition. | New York : Tiller Press, 2020.
Identifiers: LCCN 2020003484 (print) | LCCN 2020003485 (ebook) |
ISBN 9781982150082 (paperback) | ISBN 9781982150099 (ebook)
Subjects: LCSH: Acupressure.
Classification: LCC RM723.A27 B753 2020 (print) | LCC RM723.A27 (ebook) |
DDC 615.8/222–dc23
LC record available at https://lccn.loc.gov/2020003484
LC ebook record available at https://lccn.loc.gov/2020003485

ISBN 978-1-9821-5008-2
ISBN 978-1-9821-5009-9 (ebook)

To my children, Mara and Tyler,
with unconditional love

CONTENTS

HEALING

AT YOUR

FINGERTIPS

INTRODUCTION

WITH THE MODERN world perpetually running at a breakneck pace, there has never been a better time to spread the word of simple self-healing. Technology has become an inescapable part of our daily lives, and many of us find ourselves seeking a more integrated relationship between our body, mind, and spirit.

This book provides a basic introduction to some of the foundational principles of a simple and effective form of energy medicine called the Art of Jin Shin.

If you've read *The Art of Jin Shin*, you already know something about the simple and effective form of energy medicine called Jin Shin. If you've picked up this book without any prior knowledge of the subject, you will find everything you need to get started with this energy healing modality we'll be exploring. The practice has many thousands of adherents all around the world, from my New York City–based clients, to the inmates at a jail in the Indian province of Gujarat, to several hospital programs in the United States, and to the many men, women, and children who have been helped by Jin Shin Jyutsu in Japan, its birthplace.

You will find everything you need to get started within the pages that follow. And since this simple energy work involves no tools other than your own two hands, you will always be ready to relieve your aches and pains or set yourself up for a great day.

GETTING STARTED

THOUGH THE ART of Jin Shin bears some similarities to acupuncture, the practice achieves its transformative results without needles, using only a gentle touch—a methodology that translates very nicely to self-care. All you need to get started are your hands and a little bit of time and patience.

The holds in this book will grow more effective as you become a more adept reader of your body's signals. However and whenever you start, to some degree you will succeed in moving stagnant energy and restoring harmony right from the get-go, and that's part of the beauty of the Art of Jin Shin.

Each of us is endowed with the ability to balance and heal our physical, mental, and spiritual selves. Jin Shin allows us to tap into the body's innate wisdom, lifting us out of the jagged rhythms of modern life and returning our bodies to the rhythm of the universal clock. We always have the necessary tools to practice—our breath and hands—and there's no way to harm ourselves using the holds and quick fixes.

I'm happy to be able to share some of the magical quick fixes in *Healing at Your Fingertips*. The holds presented here have been literal lifesavers countless times—sometimes for a stranger on a street corner or a straphanger on a subway car, and more than once, for myself.

Many years ago I was walking down the street with my aunt Mimi, an old-school Dutch traditionalist with little interest in alternative healing practices. She was overcome with a sudden need to void her bowels, but there were no bathrooms in sight. I dug into her left lower back and the outer side of the back of her right knee, and the sense of urgency instantly vanished.

Likewise, I have had so many opportunities to use Jin Shin with strangers that I sometimes feel the universe is pushing them into my path. Maybe the same will happen to you.

I hope you enjoy the benefits of a medicine cabinet fully stocked with nature's own prescription medicine. Your friends and family are likely to love your newly acquired Jin Shin skills, too.

THE SAFETY ENERGY LOCATIONS

THE TWENTY-SIX SAFETY Energy Locations (SELs) are vital to our practice. Located on the right and left sides of the body (with twenty-six per side) and dispersed along the front and back sides, these three-inch areas, used along with the fingers and vertebrae on the spine and main center line of the body, are the primary sites for a Jin Shin treatment plan.

For a Jin Shin practitioner, the SELs are used in specific combinations to allow energy to move in the body. We use our hands to apply treatment to the SELs and other vital points in the body, gathering feedback as we work. Listening to the energy spiraling to the core of the body and back at relevant SELs, we leave our hands in place until we feel the energy harmonize. The pulses will slow, quicken, and/or steady as the client's energy comes into alignment, and other energetic cues such as excessive heat, cold, swelling and congestion, or discoloring may dissipate. Distinct from the arterial pulses, which measure the flow of blood to and from the heart, Jin Shin's energetic pulses are the result of the primal energy spiraling to the bone or the core of the body and back in response to the practitioner's touch. The need to feel a pulse quickening or slowing as the treatment takes hold is one of several reasons Jin Shin practitioners use their hands instead of needles (as in acupuncture) or other implements. The pulses give us information about which areas of the body need to be harmonized.

You may have some difficulty discerning these signals as you begin your Jin Shin self-care journey. Slow down and breathe, and with a little practice, you will soon be able to "hear" the energy pulsating through your SELs.

The following section introduces the meanings, locations, and uses of the individual Safety Energy Locations. It is intended to help you familiarize yourself with your body's energetic map as it is understood within the Art of Jin Shin. You can practice one or more holds at a time, holding a few minutes per hold.

SEL 1: The Prime Mover

Located on the inside of the knee, where the femur articulates with the tibia.

Note: This area appears in two iterations, as SEL 1 and SEL High 1.

SEL 2: Innate Knowing

Located at the crest of the hip, in the lower back area.

SEL 3: The Breath

Located at the top of the shoulder blade, between the blade and the spine.

SEL 4: The Bridge

Located at the base of the head, at the occipital ridge.

SEL 5: Regeneration

Located just beneath the anklebone at the inner ankle.

SEL 6: The Root

Located on the sole of the foot.

SEL 7: Stillness

Located on the pad of the big toe.

SEL 8: Infinity

Located on the back of the knee, on the lateral side (outside).

    Note: This point appears in two iterations, as SEL 8 and SEL Low 8.

SEL 9: Endings

Located level with the bottom of the shoulder blade, between the blade and the spine.

SEL 10: Beginnings

Located between the shoulder blade and the spine, midway down the blade.

SEL 11: Unloading

Located at the top of the shoulder, where the neck curves into the shoulder.

SEL 12: Surrender

Located midway down the neck, between the base of the head and the shoulders.

SEL 13: Creativity

Located on the middle of the chest, at the third rib.

SEL 14: Nourishment

Located at bottom of the rib cage.

SEL 15: The Joy Giver

Located in the groin area at the top of the thigh.

SEL 16: Transformation

Located just beneath the anklebone at the outer ankle.

SEL 17: Intuition

Located at the wrist joint, on the little finger side.

SEL 18: Peaceful Mind

Located on the palm side of hand, at the base of the thumb.

SEL 19: The Commander

Located in the crease of the elbow, on the thumb side.

Note: This point appears in two iterations, as SEL 19 and SEL High 19.

SEL 20: Clear Mind

Located on the forehead, just above the eyebrow.

SEL 21: Calm Mind

Located just beneath the cheekbone.

SEL 22: Exhale

Located just beneath the collarbone.

SEL 23: Fearlessness
Located on the middle of the back.

SEL 24: The Peacemaker
Located at the top of the outer foot, about midway between the little toe and the fourth toe.

SEL 25: The Regenerator
Located on the sit bones (ischium).

SEL 26: Completion
Located at the outer edge of the shoulder blade, near the armpit.

Safety Energy Locations when in harmony are close to the spine. It is our lifestyle that pulls them over to the side. Each of us is unique, and for this reason, it is important that you find your SELs and where they need to be harmonized.

CHOOSING LEFT OR RIGHT SIDES FOR QUICK FIXES AND FINGER HOLDS

How to decide which side of the body to treat? Go to the side that seems to have a more pressing need, where the relevant SELs feel more tender or full, while keeping in mind that the energy will always find its way. Usually reversing the instructions from left to right will simply help the other side of the body. Some of the holds where arms are crossed or holding mirror-image positions treat both sides of the body equally. In a few cases, however, where noted, you'll find that one side of the flow harmonizes one kind of symptom, while the other tends to the opposite symptom (as in the case of constipation and diarrhea).

Along with instructions for the quick fixes, I've also included an even quicker alternate option in the form of a finger hold.

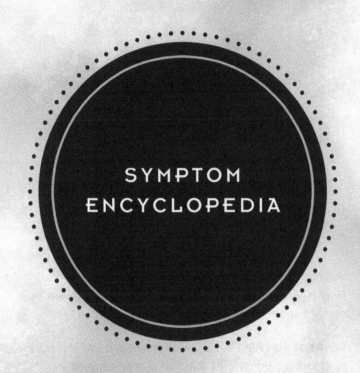

SYMPTOM
ENCYCLOPEDIA

ALLERGIES
(RING FINGER)

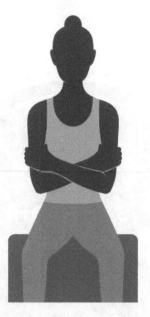

Place right hand on left upper arm (SEL High 19) and left hand on right upper arm (SEL High 19).

WHAT IT HELPS: Clears the chestline and harmonizes the lung energy, aiding with seasonal allergy symptoms such as runny nose, wheezing, and chest congestion.

ANGER
(MIDDLE FINGER)

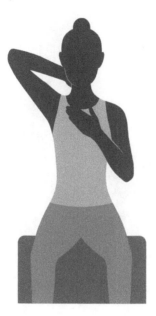

Place right hand on left base of head (SEL 4) and left hand below right collarbone (SEL 22).

WHAT IT HELPS: This quickie allows anger to melt away. Holding the middle finger—the very same finger many of us tend to raise when we are angry—while practicing specialized, abdominal breathing is also great for temper tantrums.

ARTHRITIS
(LITTLE FINGER)

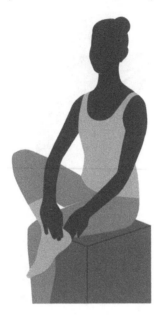

Place right hand beneath inside of right anklebone (SEL 5) and left hand beneath outer right anklebone (SEL 16).

WHAT IT HELPS: Pain and inflammation in the joints, along with deep bodily fatigue.

ASTHMA
(RING FINGER)

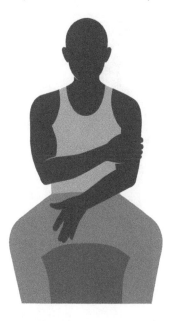

Place right hand on left upper arm (SEL High 19) and left hand on inside of right thigh (SEL High 1).

WHAT IT HELPS: This quickie helps to open up the lungs and clear the chest. The SEL on the upper arm opens up the chestline, while the SEL on the thigh creates an escape route for the congestion.

AUTOIMMUNE PROJECTS (PALM)

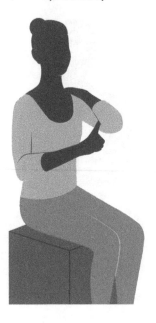

Place right index finger in left elbow crease (SEL 19) and left hand on top of left shoulder (SELs 11 and 3).

WHAT IT HELPS: This quickie helps conditions such as Lyme disease, lupus, multiple sclerosis, and rheumatoid arthritis, and balances the lymphatic system.

BABIES
(THUMB)

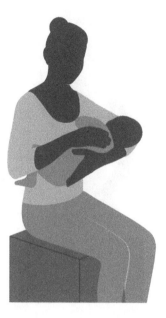

Place right hand on bottom of left shoulder blade (SELs 9 and 26) and left hand on right lower back (SEL 2).

WHAT IT HELPS: An all-purpose flow for babies (crying, upset stomach, etc.), the hold complements the natural breast-feeding position, making it a perfect option for multitasking! Hold SEL 26, at the outer edge of the shoulder blade, with your thumb and reach to the bottom of the shoulder blade, between blade and spine, SEL 9, with your fingers. Fittingly, the complementary finger hold is the thumb, which babies instinctively suckle for some self-soothing Jin Shin.

BACK PAIN
(INDEX FINGER)

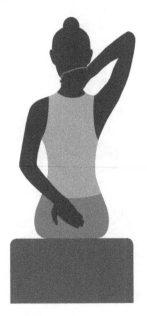

Place right hand on left middle of neck (SEL 12) and left hand on tailbone.

WHAT IT HELPS: This quickie eases back pain, which is often related to fear.

BED-WETTING
(INDEX FINGER)

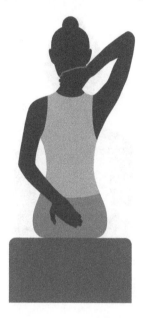

Place right hand on left middle of neck (SEL 12) and left hand on tailbone.

WHAT IT HELPS: Opens up the bladder line to help balance the containment or free flow of bladder function. Bed-wetting is often related to fear.

BLADDER INFECTION
(INDEX FINGER)

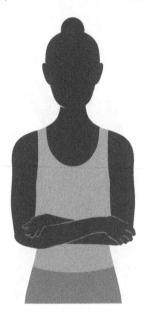

Place right hand at crease of left elbow (SEL 19) and left hand at crease of right elbow (SEL 19).

WHAT IT HELPS: The self-help hold for SEL 9, which is located in a difficult-to-reach location between the shoulder blades, the elbow points help clear up bladder infections.

BLOOD PRESSURE
(INDEX FINGER)

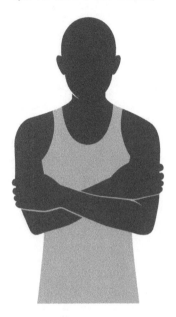

Place right hand on left upper arm (SEL High 19) and left hand on right upper arm (SEL High 19).

WHAT IT HELPS: This quickie harmonizes the heart function energy and opens up the chestline, balancing the speed and strength of your blood circulation.

BONES
(LITTLE FINGER)

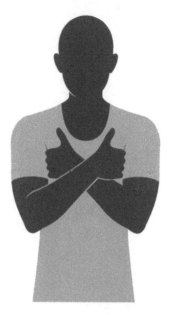

As if giving yourself a hug, reach beneath the left armpit to place right fingertips at the outer edge of left shoulder blade (SEL 26), resting right thumb beneath left collarbone (SEL 22). Mirror these positions on the left, placing left fingertips on the outer edge of right shoulder blade (SEL 26) and left thumb beneath right collarbone (SEL 22).

WHAT IT HELPS: The position at the outer edge of the shoulder blade helps to strengthen the skeletal system and bones, while the location beneath the collarbone helps the thyroid, which is responsible for calcium absorption.

BRAIN
(MIDDLE FINGER)

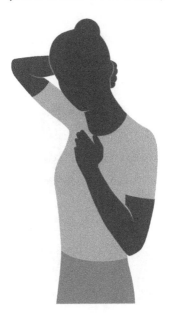

Place right hand on left base of head (SEL 4) and left hand below right collarbone (SEL 22).

WHAT IT HELPS: Helpful for any issues involving the brain, this quickie is a useful tool for anyone recovering from a concussion or for brain development.

BREAST

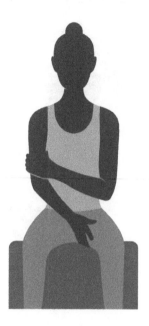

Place right hand on left inside thigh (SEL High 1) and left hand on right upper arm (SEL High 19).

WHAT IT HELPS: Any accumulations in the breasts. Applying this flow three times a day for twenty minutes over a three-week period may clear any breast project. Apply to the upper arm on the same side as the project, with the SEL on the thigh opposite the side in need.

BREATHING
(RING FINGER)

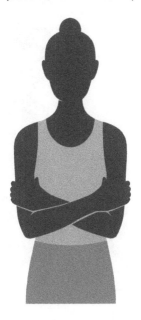

Place right hand on left upper arm (SEL High 19) and left hand on right upper arm (SEL High 19).

WHAT IT HELPS: This quickie will open up the chestline and help the lungs, allowing for easy, deeper breathing while relieving any chest congestion.

BURNS
(THUMB)

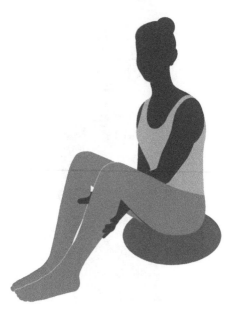

Place right hand on left calf and left hand on right calf, fingers pointing down and palming the calves.

WHAT IT HELPS: Repairing burn trauma; helpful as first aid for minor burns and for patients recovering from medical treatment for serious burns.

CHEST
(INDEX FINGER)

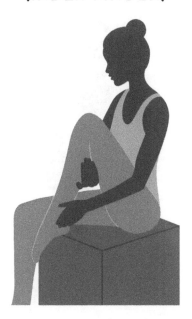

Place right hand on back of knee, on lateral side (outside) (SEL 8), and left hand just beneath anklebone at the outer ankle (SEL 16).

WHAT IT HELPS: This special little flow helps to open up the chest, allowing stuck energy to move down and facilitating deep breathing while aiding with issues such as asthma, chronic cough, and bronchitis.

CHOKING
(THUMB)

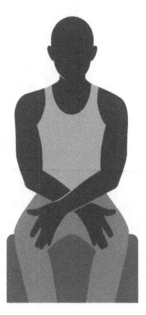

Place right hand inside left knee, where the femur articulates with the tibia (SEL 1), and left hand inside right knee (SEL 1).

WHAT IT HELPS: An adjunct to the Heimlich maneuver, this emergency first aid hold will open up the throat and bring up the stuck piece of food or object causing the obstruction. When using in an emergency situation, apply strongly, adding much more pressure to the SEL than you normally would when practicing Jin Shin.

CHOLESTEROL
(INDEX FINGER)

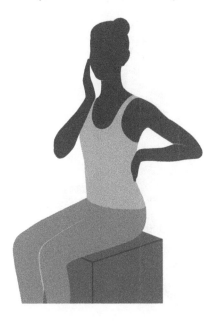

Place right hand beneath right cheekbone (SEL 21) and left hand on left middle of back (SEL 23).

WHAT IT HELPS: This quickie aids in the flushing of cholesterol by facilitating the exhale and aiding in the letting go of any accumulations in the body.

COLDS
(ALL FINGERS)

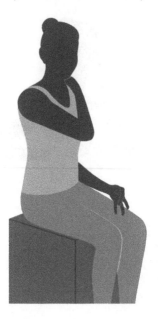

Place right hand on top of left shoulder between blade and spine (SEL 3), then form a ring with left pad of thumb over each left fingernail, beginning with the little finger.

WHAT IT HELPS: The key to the immune system, the location at the top of the shoulder blade bolsters your body's ability to fight off and recover from ailments like the common cold, while holding each of the fingers optimizes all of the organ functions. Apply to the side of the SEL that feels tighter (more congested) to you.

CONSTIPATION
(INDEX FINGER)

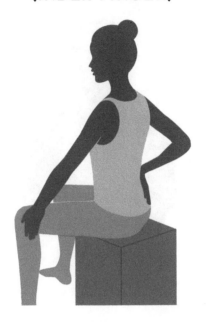

Place right hand at right crest of hip, lower back (SEL 2), and left hand on left back of knee, on lateral side (outside) (SEL 8).

WHAT IT HELPS: Works on the pelvic line, allowing your abdomen and intestines to relax and encouraging elimination. Reverse for diarrhea, page 37.

COUGH
(INDEX FINGER)

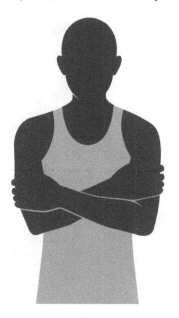

Place right hand on left upper arm (SEL High 19) and left hand on right upper arm (SEL High 19).

WHAT IT HELPS: Holding the upper arms connects into the lung function pathway, helping to clear the lungs and loosening up excess phlegm so it can be released by coughing. You can place your fingers on the backs of the upper arms, thumbs on the insides of the upper arms, in order to cover additional energetic ground.

DEPRESSION
(INDEX FINGER)

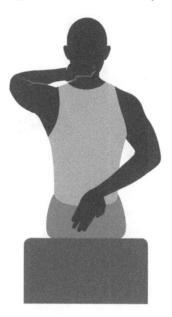

Place right hand on tailbone and left hand on right middle of neck (SEL 12).

WHAT IT HELPS: This quickie brings the energy down out of the face and head. In dealing with recurring emotional and psychological issues, moving energy that is stuck in the head down to below the waist is essential.

DIABETES
(THUMB)

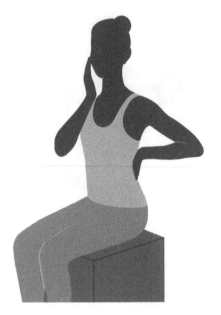

Place right hand beneath right cheekbone (SEL 21) and left hand on left middle of back (SEL 23).

WHAT IT HELPS: This quickie helps balance the sugars in your digestive system and blood, harmonizing digestion on both the physical and mental plane.

DIARRHEA
(INDEX FINGER)

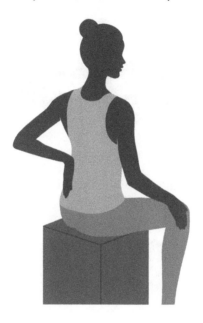

Place right hand on right back of knee, on the lateral side (outside) (SEL 8) and left hand on left lower back at crest of hip (SEL 2).

WHAT IT HELPS: All SELs on the left side of the body help to "build," as does the location on the lower back, which will help reduce looseness during bowel movements. The location on the outside of the right knee will help to clear the pelvic area and abdomen, harmonizing elimination. Reverse for constipation, page 33.

DIZZINESS
(PALM)

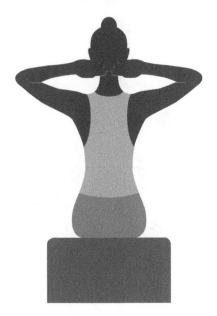

Place right hand on right base of head (SEL 4) and left hand on left base of head (SEL 4).

WHAT IT HELPS: Bridges the gap between consciousness and unconsciousness or the spiritual and physical realm. The left side of the location helps the head, while the right tends to the body.

EARACHE
(LITTLE FINGER)

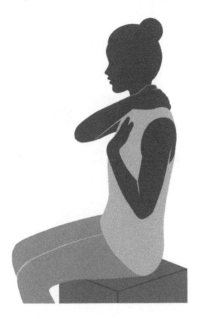

Place right hand on top of left shoulder (SEL 11) and left hand below right middle of chest (SEL 13).

WHAT IT HELPS: This hold circulates energy through the ear, helping to relieve earaches. To ease discomfort while flying, hold the little fingers until you feel your ears pop.

EATING DISORDER: ANOREXIA
(INDEX FINGER)

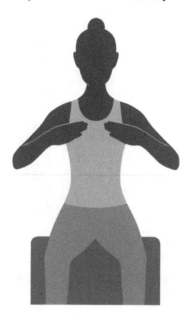

Place right hand on right middle of chest (SEL 13) and left hand in the same spot on left middle of chest (SEL 13).

WHAT IT HELPS: Because anorexia provides a false sense of control, it is frequently used as a form of emotional suppression. A key location for emotional balance, this area on the chestline helps promote the free flow of feelings while also balancing appetite.

EATING DISORDER: BULIMIA (THUMB)

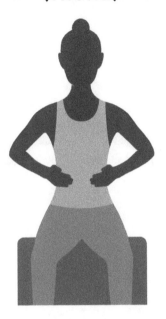

Place right hand at right bottom of rib cage (SEL 14) and left hand at left bottom of rib cage (SEL 14).

WHAT IT HELPS: Helping to balance the waistline, which is responsible for our digestive system and for gaining "control in our life," a function of the mind related to waistline projects. When harmonizing these locations, we can let go of the false sense of control afforded by destructive habits such as bulimia.

EMOTIONAL TRAUMA
(INDEX FINGER)

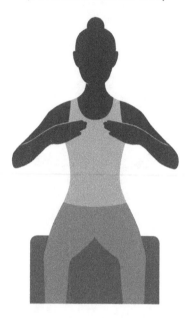

Place right hand on right middle of chest (SEL 13) and left hand on left middle of chest (SEL 13).

WHAT IT HELPS: Fostering emotional balance and harmony while nurturing our connection to spirit, these points help the exhale move all the way down to the toes, allowing us to let go of stuck emotions.

ENDOMETRIOSIS
(INDEX FINGER)

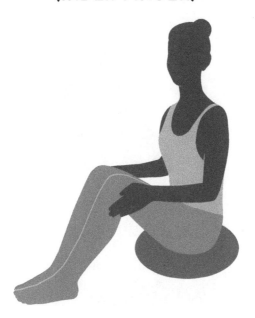

Place right hand on back of right knee, on the lateral side (outside) (SEL 8) and left hand on back of left knee, on the lateral side (outside) (SEL 8).

WHAT IT HELPS: Dissolving accumulations as well as assisting with elimination and muscular conditions, this hold helps any projects related to the pelvic area. Used during childbirth, the hold can even open up the pelvic cavity.

EYES
(MIDDLE FINGER)

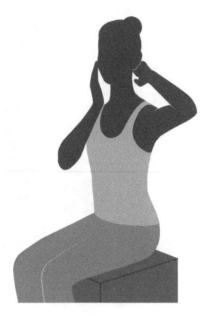

Place right hand beneath right cheekbone (SEL 21) and left hand on left base of head (SEL 4).

WHAT IT HELPS: The point on the base of the head allows energy to ascend into the head, while the point on the cheekbone moves the energy down the front, clearing the head.

FATIGUE
(PALM)

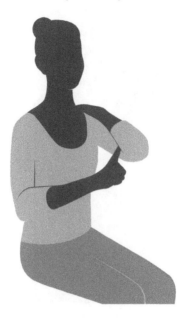

Place right index finger in left elbow crease (SEL 19) and left hand on top of left shoulder (SELs 11 and 3).

WHAT IT HELPS: This hold helps rev up slow-moving energy, that sense of "drag," by harmonizing the lymphatic system. When overuse and abuse of the body build up fatigue, you may feel it as a fullness or accumulation in the elbow creases (SEL 19).

FEAR
(INDEX FINGER)

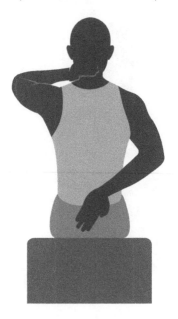

Place right hand on tailbone and left hand on right middle of neck (SEL 12).

WHAT IT HELPS: This hold helps harmonize anxiety and fear, which the Art of Jin Shin considers to be a main cause of imbalance in the body.

FEET
(MIDDLE FINGER)

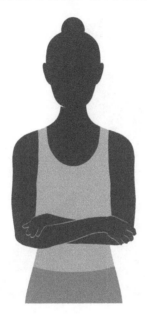

Place right hand at crease of left elbow (SEL 19) and left hand at crease of right elbow (SEL 19).

WHAT IT HELPS: "The Nines," located in a hard-to-reach spot at the bottom of the shoulder blades, are the helpers for any project related to the feet—bunions, corns, spurs, dropped feet, foot injuries, and tired, achy feet. If you can reach your own, feel free to do so. Otherwise, practice this quick hold.

FEVER AND FLU
(ALL FINGERS)

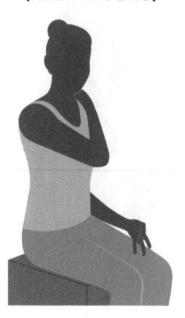

Place right hand on top of left shoulder, between the blade and the spine (SEL 3), then form a ring with left pad of thumb over each left fingernail, beginning with the little finger.

WHAT IT HELPS: The location on the top of the shoulder blade boosts the immune system, while the fingers connect to the organ flows, helping the entire body.

FOCUS
(MIDDLE FINGER)

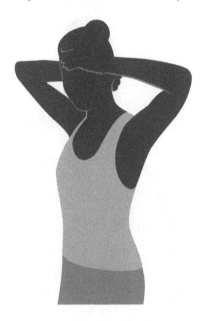

Place right hand on left middle of neck (SEL 12) and left hand on right middle of the forehead (SEL 20).

WHAT IT HELPS: This quickie will clear the mind and help with focus. (Ever notice when you forget something, you touch your forehead to help jog your memory? That's an instinctive use of SEL 20. Nice job!)

GAS
(INDEX FINGER)

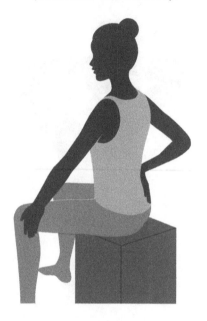

Place right hand at right crest of hip, lower back (SEL 2), and left hand on left back of knee, on lateral side (outside) (SEL 8).

WHAT IT HELPS: Harmonizing the pelvic and abdominal areas, this hold will help you release excess gas. If the discomfort is concentrated on one side, start with the opposite knee and move the sacral hand to the side where the discomfort is. Babies with digestive issues tend to respond well to this hold.

GRIEF
(RING FINGER)

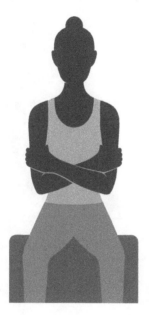

Place right hand on left upper arm (SEL High 19) and left hand on right upper arm (SEL High 19).

WHAT IT HELPS: Clears the chestline, helping to open the heart and lung energy and allowing us to move through feelings of grief.

HEADACHES
(MIDDLE FINGER)

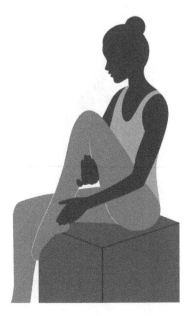

Place right hand on back of left knee, on the lateral side (outside) (SEL 8), and left hand just beneath outer left anklebone (SEL 16).

WHAT IT HELPS: This quickie brings the energy down from the head to the toes.

HEARTBURN AND INDIGESTION (THUMB)

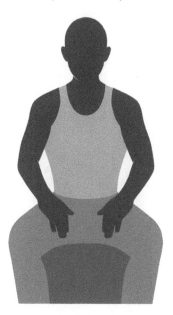

Place right hand on right upper thigh (SEL High 1) and left hand on left upper thigh (SEL High 1).

WHAT IT HELPS: We often hold our upper inner thighs instinctively after a large meal to naturally boost our digestion, and in this hold we add some conscious breathing to bolster the position's effects. Stress, one potential cause for heartburn, can cause the energy to reverse and travel up the front of the body rather than down, a phenomenon countered by this hold. You may cross your hands if that is more comfortable. For an ultra-quickie, hold the thumb to balance acidity in the body.

HEART PALPITATIONS
(LITTLE FINGER)

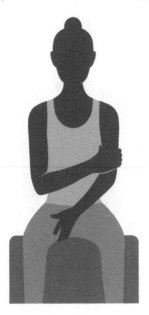

Place right hand on left upper arm (SEL High 19) and left hand on right upper thigh (SEL High 1).

WHAT IT HELPS: The position on the left upper arm helps the heart, and the location on the right upper thigh gives the energy an escape route, helping congested energy clear out of the chest. When acute, dig in to the little finger strongly. Note: There's no harm in reversing this flow, but the side demonstrated above will be most effective.

HICCUPS
(PALM)

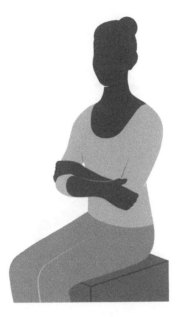

Place right hand in crease of left elbow (SEL 19) and left hand in crease of right elbow (SEL 19).

WHAT IT HELPS: Clears the waistline and relaxes the diaphragm muscle from the spasm that is the cause for hiccups. Helpful for kids with hiccups, too!

HORMONAL BALANCE
(RING FINGER)

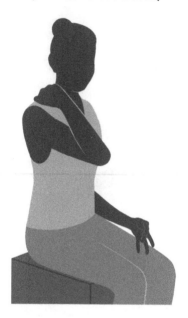

Place right hand on top of right shoulder (SEL 11) and form a ring with pad of left thumb over left ring fingernail.

WHAT IT HELPS: This quickie helps harmonize any hormonal imbalances for men and women of all ages. Helpful for reproductive issues in both men and women, as well as for menopausal issues. Helpful during pregnancy and for postnatal self-care, when hormones are raging through the body.

HYPERACTIVITY
(LITTLE FINGER)

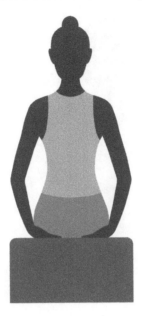

Place right and left hands under the sit bones (SEL 25).

WHAT IT HELPS: Children naturally sit on their hands to re-charge their batteries and ground themselves; a pose that can help you calm and regenerate your entire body.

IMMUNE SYSTEM
(THUMB)

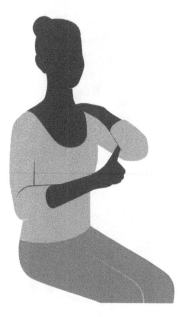

Place right index finger in left elbow crease (SEL 19) and left hand on top of left shoulder (SELs 11 and 3).

WHAT IT HELPS: This hold includes SEL 3, the key to the immune system. Helpful for any immune conditions falling under the medical label of "fatigue syndrome," including viruses that yield symptoms of extreme tiredness. Stimulating the movement of the lymphatic system as well as swollen glands, it's a great option for times when there is no clear diagnosis but you know something is going on in your body.

INDIGESTION
(THUMB)

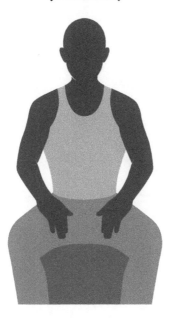

Place right hand on right upper thigh (SEL High 1) and left hand on left upper thigh (SEL High 1).

WHAT IT HELPS: We often hold our upper inner thighs instinctively after a large meal to naturally boost our digestion, and in this hold we add some conscious breathing to bolster the position's effects. Stress, one potential cause for heartburn, can cause the energy to reverse and travel up the front of the body rather than down, a phenomenon countered by this hold. You may cross your hands if that is more comfortable. For an ultra-quickie, hold the thumb to balance acidity in the body.

INSOMNIA
(THUMB)

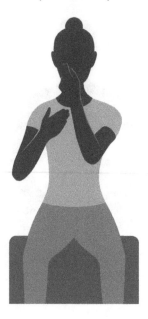

Place right hand beneath right collarbone (SEL 22) and left hand beneath right cheekbone (SEL 21).

WHAT IT HELPS: This quickie helps relax the mind and calm the nervous system for a peaceful sleep.

IRRITABILITY
(MIDDLE FINGER)

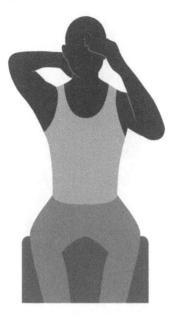

Place right hand on right middle of neck (SEL 12) and left hand on left forehead, just above the eyebrow (SEL 20).

WHAT IT HELPS: Brings peace of mind as it harmonizes anger and frustration.

ITCHING
(THUMB)

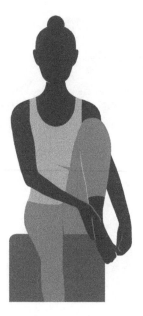

Place right hand on sole of left foot (SEL 6) and left hand on left little toe.

WHAT IT HELPS: This hold will help any itchy skin surface issue you may have, such as hives, burns, allergic reactions, or acne. The hold as pictured works on the left side of the body; for itching on the right side, reverse.

JAUNDICE
(MIDDLE FINGER)

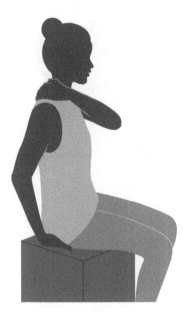

Place right hand on right sit bone (SEL 25) and left hand on top of right shoulder (SEL 11).

WHAT IT HELPS: Helpful with conditions of jaundice (a yellowish tone in the skin) related to the energetic needs of liver function energy. Performed as demonstrated on the right side (where the liver is located), this quickie helps us with the exhale, revitalizing the energy down the front of the body as it harmonizes the energy of the liver. It's okay to reverse this quickie, though it will be more effective on the right.

JAW TIGHTNESS
(INDEX FINGER)

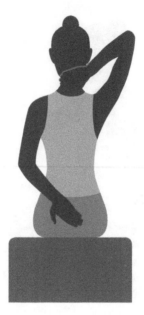

Place right hand on middle of neck (SEL 12) and left hand on tailbone.

WHAT IT HELPS: Relieves clenching of teeth causing jaw tightness, often occurring during sleep.

JET LAG
(ALL FINGERS AND PALM)

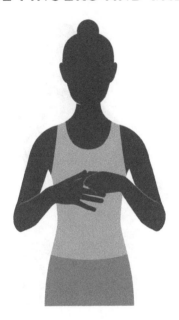

Hold each finger individually for about two minutes or until you feel a regular, harmonious pulsation in the fingers.

WHAT IT HELPS: Harmonizes the body to the circadian rhythm as you energize each organ function. Help ward off jet lag before it hits by administering during long plane trips—hold your fingers when taking off, fold your hands while sleeping, and repeat before landing.

JOY
(LITTLE FINGER)

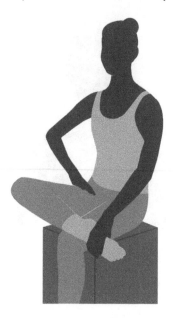

Place right hand on top of right thigh at groin area (SEL 15) and left thumb on sole of right foot (SEL 6).

WHAT IT HELPS: Allows us to exhale so we can bring in joy!

MENOPAUSE
(RING FINGER)

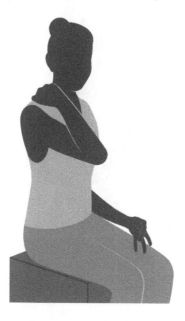

Place right hand on top of right shoulder (SEL 11) and form a ring with pad of left thumb over left ring fingernail.

WHAT IT HELPS: This quickie helps harmonize any hormonal imbalances for men and women of all ages. Helpful for reproductive issues in both men and women, as well as for menopausal issues. Helpful during pregnancy and for postnatal self-care, when hormones are raging through the body.

MENSTRUAL CRAMPS
(INDEX FINGER)

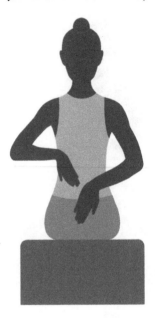

Place right hand on sacrum and left hand on left middle-lower back (SEL 23).

WHAT IT HELPS: The location on the sacrum helps to clear pelvic discomfort. In combination with the location on the middle-lower back (a great spot for hormonal balance), it also works on stomach cramps due to menstruation.

MOTION SICKNESS
(BACK OF WRIST)

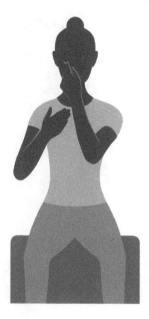

Place right hand beneath right collarbone (SEL 22) and left hand beneath right cheekbone (SEL 21).

WHAT IT HELPS: Motion sickness and nausea correspond to the sensation of energy getting stuck in the waistline, unable to descend. This hold will help release SEL 14 (located at the bottom of the ribs) and allow energy to descend.

NASAL CONGESTION
(INDEX FINGER)

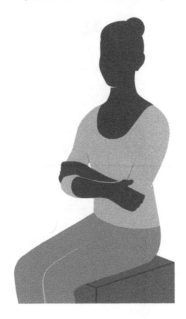

Place right hand in crease of left elbow (SEL 19) and left hand in crease of right elbow (SEL 19).

WHAT IT HELPS: "The Nines," located in a hard-to-reach spot at the bottom of the shoulder blades, clear nasal congestion. If you find them difficult to reach, you can hold the elbow points as demonstrated. Harmonizing kidney energy, which flows through the nostrils and nasal passageways, the hold will clear any nasal congestion.

NAUSEA
(BACK OF WRIST)

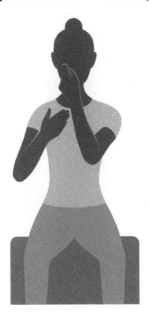

Place right hand beneath right collarbone (SEL 22) and left hand beneath right cheekbone (SEL 21).

WHAT IT HELPS: Motion sickness and nausea correspond to the sensation of energy getting stuck in the waistline, unable to descend. This hold will help release SEL 14 (located at the bottom of the ribs) and allow energy to descend.

NOSEBLEEDS
(INDEX FINGER)

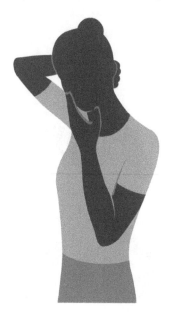

Place right hand on left high back of neck close to spine (SELs 4 and 12) and left hand beneath right cheekbone close to nose (SEL 21).

WHAT IT HELPS: Kidney energy, accessed through SELs 4 and 12, can be a cause for nosebleeds if blood stagnates in the muscles alongside the spine.

OSTEOPOROSIS
(LITTLE FINGER)

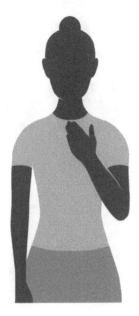

Place left fingertips in V of neck, where collarbone connects to sternum.

WHAT IT HELPS: Resolving congestion in this area enables the body to absorb calcium. Check right and left side of V for fullness and/or tenderness at area of congestion.

PARKINSON'S-LIKE CONDITIONS (MIDDLE FINGER)

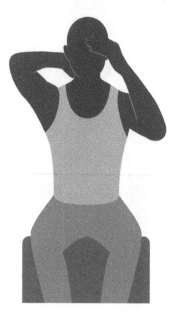

Place right hand on right middle of neck (SEL 12) and left hand on left middle of forehead (SEL 20).

WHAT IT HELPS: This hold is helpful for any tremor condition in the head and body, Parkinson's included. You may find fullness or tightness a little bit sideways from the center of the neck; follow the congestion.

PSORIASIS
(INDEX FINGER)

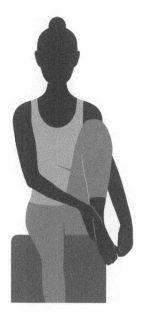

Place right hand on sole of left foot (SEL 6) and left hand on left little toe.

WHAT IT HELPS: This hold will help any itchy skin surface issue you may have, such as hives, burns, allergic reactions, or acne. The hold as pictured works on the left side of the body; for itching on the right side, reverse.

SADNESS
(RING FINGER)

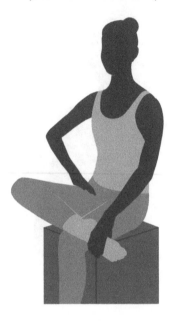

Place right hand on top of right thigh at groin area (SEL 15) and left thumb on sole of left foot (SEL 6).

WHAT IT HELPS: Hold these points to bring laughter, joy, and balance into your life.

SHOCK, EMOTIONAL
(INDEX FINGER)

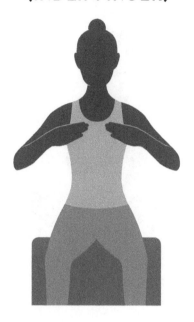

Place right hand on right middle of chest (SEL 13) and left hand on left middle of chest (SEL 13).

WHAT IT HELPS: Fostering emotional balance and harmony while nurturing our connection to spirit, these points help the exhale move all the way down to the toes, allowing us to let go of stuck emotions.

SHOCK, PHYSICAL
(LITTLE FINGER)

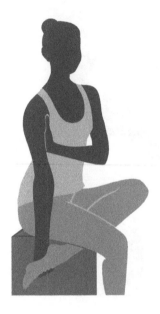

Place right hand at top of outer left foot midway between little toe and the fourth toe (SEL 24). Place left hand at outer edge of the right shoulder blade, near armpit.

WHAT IT HELPS: This quickie calms and grounds chaos on a physical and emotional level. It helps the core of our being.

SHOULDER PAIN
(INDEX FINGER)

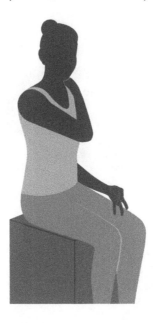

Place right hand on top of left shoulder (SELs 11 and 3) and form a ring by placing left pad of thumb over left ring finger-nail.

WHAT IT HELPS: The location on the shoulder allows regional muscular tension to release, while holding the ring finger helps the lungs and breathing, opening any congested areas. Muscular tension is often connected to issues in the breath.

SINUS
(INDEX FINGER)

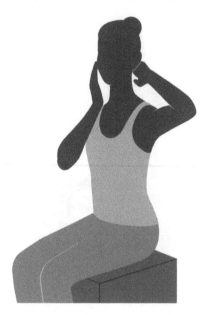

Place right hand beneath right cheekbone close to nose (SEL 21) and left hand on left back of neck (SELs 4 and 12).

WHAT IT HELPS: This quickie helps to open the sinuses and clear the nasal passages so we can breathe freely. Stay closer to the midline on SEL 21 to open up the sinuses.

SKIN
(THUMB)

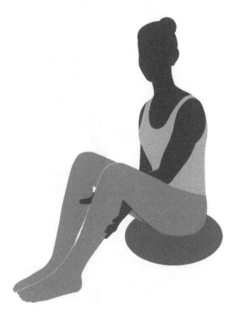

Place right hand on left calf and left hand on right calf, fingers pointing down and palming the calves.

WHAT IT HELPS: Repairing burn trauma; helpful as first aid for minor burns and for patients recovering from medical treatment for serious burns.

SORE THROAT
(LITTLE FINGER)

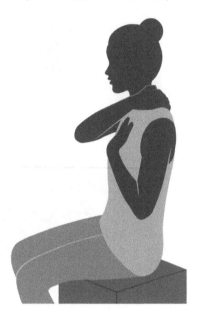

Place right hand on top of left shoulder (SEL 11) and left hand on right middle of chest (SEL 13).

WHAT IT HELPS: These locations harmonize a sore throat. To choose the optimal side on which to practice, palpate both sides of SEL 13, at the middle of chest, until you find a spot that feels tender—that will be the side of choice to use for this quickie. When in doubt, just do both!

SPINE
(PALM)

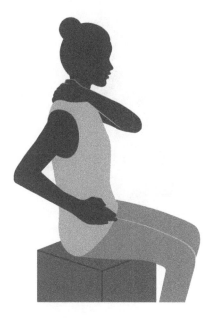

Place right hand on right upper thigh at the groin area (SEL 15) and left hand on top of right shoulder close to spine (SEL 11).

WHAT IT HELPS: Any issue on the spine can be traced to an energetic cause on the front of the body. That is why we hold SEL 15, allowing the energy to move down the front of the body so it is able to flow up the back.

STOMACH CRAMPS
(THUMB)

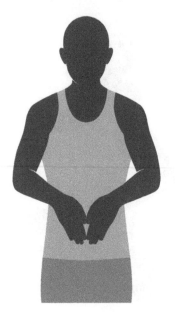

1 When pain is scattered, place both hands on stomach, fingertips pointing down, thumbs together.

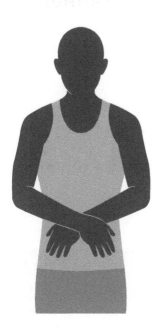

2 When pain is localized, cross both hands on stomach, fingertips pointing down, thumbs apart.

WHAT IT HELPS: Holding the thumbs together will bring the energy in toward the center of the belly, an excellent hold for general stomach pain without a single, precise location. If the pain is in one particular spot, the energy needs to be dispersed, so cross your hands, one over the other, bringing the thumbs apart.

STRESS
(THUMB)

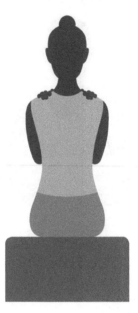

Place right hand on top of right shoulder (SEL 11) and left hand on top of left shoulder (SEL 11).

WHAT IT HELPS: "The Elevens" are the SELs where we tend to pile up all of our stress, whether work related, relationship oriented, or due to what we call "burdens of life." We also call these points "the hub," and many of us store an excess of muscular tension here. Exhale as you hold your Elevens, and let go.

TENNIS ELBOW
(INDEX FINGER)

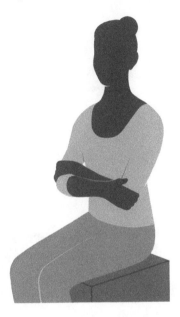

Place right hand in crease of left elbow (SEL 19) and left hand in crease of right elbow (SEL) 19.

WHAT IT HELPS: Relieve pain and inflammation in the elbow by holding the tender spot.

THYROID
(MIDDLE FINGER)

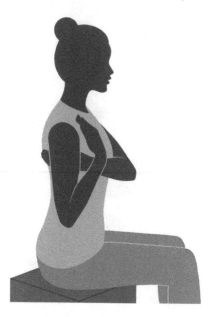

Place right hand beneath right collarbone (SEL 22) and left hand at outer edge of right shoulder blade (SEL 26).

WHAT IT HELPS: This hold will open up your chest area while boosting thyroid function. Reverse for equal attention to both sides or check for congestion where the neck meets the shoulder, and apply the hold to the side where you notice a fullness.

TINNITUS
(RING FINGER)

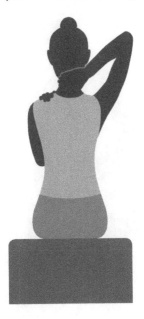

Place right hand on left middle of neck (SEL 12) and left hand on top of left shoulder (SEL 11).

WHAT IT HELPS: This hold helps ringing in the ears. Sometimes caused by emotional stress, the condition can also occur in people over the age of sixty-five.

TOOTHACHE
(INDEX FINGER)

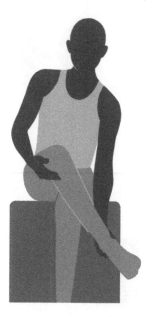

For a toothache on the left side, place right hand on right back of knee, on the lateral side (outside) (SEL 8), and left hand just beneath outer right anklebone (SEL16).

WHAT IT HELPS: Helping the large intestine energy, which flows through the gum line, this hold is very dynamic and useful for tooth infections and can help speed up healing after dental surgery.

WELL-BEING
(PALM)

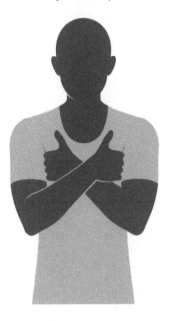

As if giving yourself a hug, reach beneath the left armpit to place right fingertips on outer left bottom of shoulder blade (SEL 26), resting right thumb below left collarbone (SEL 22). Mirror these positions on the left, placing left fingertips on outer right bottom of shoulder blade (SEL 26) and left thumb below right collarbone (SEL 22).

WHAT IT HELPS: The hold we call "the Big Hug" helps the total being, working on the exhale (SEL 22 helps us to exhale) and inhale (SEL 26 helps us to inhale) for complete energetic harmony.

ABOUT THE AUTHOR

ALEXIS BRINK is the head of Jin Shin Institute in New York City and has been a practitioner of the Art of Jin Shin since 1991. She is a licensed massage therapist and interfaith minister and has taught self-help classes and workshops in New York City as well as in different countries for many years. She has also taught Jin Shin in hospitals to medical professionals and to teachers and their students in the public school system.

This energy healing modality has not been given the attention it deserves, and Alexis has made it her personal life's journey to introduce the Art of Jin Shin to the world. Jin Shin Institute was entrusted to her by Pamela Markarian Smith in 2015. Today Jin Shin Institute, under Alexis's guidance, offers a comprehensive curriculum to a new generation of practitioners and teachers. She is creating an open and welcoming community and hopes the Art of Jin Shin will continue to spread worldwide. Visit her at jinshininstitute.com